Nutrition in Minority Groups: Asians and Afro-Caribbeans in the United Kingdom

A briefing paper prepared for health professionals by the Health Education Authority

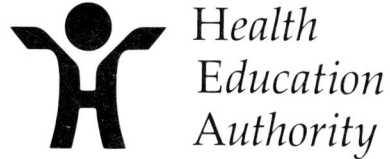

Contents

Introduction	1
Background: Asians and Afro-Caribbeans in the UK	2
Dietary patterns, practices and trends	5
The Asian community: religious and cultural traditions	5
The Afro-Caribbean community: religious and cultural traditions	11
Nutritional implications	14
Pregnant women	14
Infants and children	15
Adults	18
Conclusions	22
Further reading	24

The HEA would like to acknowledge the work of Usha Letchumanan and Jane Thomas in developing this briefing paper. The HEA is also grateful for the useful comments from Martha Annaan, Moya de Wet, Rekha Naidu, Dr Paul McKeigue and Leena Sevak.

© Health Education Authority, 1991

Reprinted 1992

ISBN 1 85448 251 3

Introduction

The Asian and Afro-Caribbean communities represent the largest minority ethnic groups in the UK. In view of concern about nutrition-related health problems, the HEA commissioned this briefing paper in an attempt to bring together the available information on a number of key questions:

- What are the cultural food beliefs and eating patterns of Afro-Caribbeans and Asians in Britain?

- What are the pressures on these communities to change from traditional dietary patterns and to what extent do beliefs and eating habits vary between generations?

- What evidence is available about the nutritional status of members of these communities?

- What are the critical areas for the practical application of health promotion?

Background: Asians and Afro-Caribbeans in the UK

Large-scale migration from the West Indies to the UK began in the late 1950s and early 1960s in response to post-war labour shortages. In recent years the term 'Afro-Caribbean' has been adopted to refer collectively to these people of African descent who came from many islands scattered across the Caribbean.

They were followed in the late 1950s and early 1960s by immigrants from India and Pakistan (later Bangladesh and Pakistan) and in the early 1970s by East African Asians. In the UK 'Asian' is generally taken to refer to all those people whose origins are from the pre-1947 Indian sub-continent, i.e. India, Pakistan and Bangladesh, including those who have migrated via East Africa. These two groups, Asians and Afro-Caribbeans, represent the largest minority ethnic communities in the UK; in 1985 it was estimated that 1% of the total UK population was of Afro-Caribbean origin and 2.3% of Asian origin. (1.4% Indian, 0.7% Pakistani and 0.2% Bangladeshi). Many of these people were born in this country, as Table 1 shows.

Although legislation now strictly limits the number of new Commonwealth immigrants, the sex and age structure of these communities means that population growth is relatively rapid. Population projections suggest that by 1991, 5% of the UK population will be of Asian or Afro-Caribbean origin.

As economic migrants, these groups were attracted to areas of the country with employment opportunities, often created by movement of the Caucasian population out of these areas. This has often resulted in concentrations in inner city areas, with attendant problems of poor housing and overcrowding. In 1977 nearly three-quarters of Asians and 80% of Afro-Caribbeans were living in the conurbations of the seven Metropolitan counties, with especially large numbers in Greater London. Since that time the Asian popula-

Table 1 *Population by ethnic origin and age, 1986–1988*

Ethnic origin	\multicolumn{5}{c}{Percentage in each age group}	Total all ages (thousands)	Percentage UK born
	0–15	16–29	30–44	45–59	60+		
White	20	22	20	17	21	51,333	96
West Indian or Guyanese	25	33	15	19	7	521	53
Indian	31	27	24	13	5	745	37
Pakistani	43	25	18	12	2	404	46
Bangladeshi	50	21	14	14	1	111	32

Source: Central Statistical Office. *Social Trends* 20. HMSO 1990

tions have grown in the Lancashire textile towns, while the distribution of the Afro-Caribbean population has remained fairly static.

A number of surveys suggest that members of these groups tend to occupy the lower socio-economic strata and suffer from disproportionately high unemployment rates. When in employment they tend to be concentrated in low-waged service sectors and unemployment may be 60–100% higher than among equally qualified Caucasians. The influence of socio-economic and environmental factors on individual health status has been well documented and needs to be taken into account when considering the specific area of nutrition.

Dietary patterns, practices and trends

Dietary practices vary greatly between different minority ethnic groups, as well as between members of each community. Some of these differences have been documented. However, at present there is still very little information available about the extent and nature of changes occurring, particularly amongst young people born in this country.

The Asian community: religious and cultural traditions

Eating habits vary greatly within the Asian community as a result of religious and cultural influences. Although religion plays a major role in determining dietary practices, the vast area from which this community has originated also means that there is considerable variation in the use of foods and styles of cooking even within the same religious grouping. The influence of regional variation can be seen in Table 2. For example, Moslems from Pakistan usually do not eat much fish, in contrast to Moslems from Bangladesh. While Hindus from the Punjab use ghee (clarified butter) as their main fat, those who come from Gujarat are more likely to use groundnut or mustard oil. Groups who have migrated via another country, such as Uganda, may show additional differences as a result.

Hindus

The majority of Hindus in the UK come from the Gujarat areas of India. Many are well educated and have achieved considerable economic success, but in certain communities the older generation work primarily in the low paid and declining textile industry and often have poor skills in English and low educational attainment. Orthodox Hindus adhere to a doctrine of non-violence and additionally regard the cow as a sacred animal. Consequently many are vegetarian and even among the non-vegetarians beef is not generally eaten, although they may eat mutton, poultry, fish and eggs. Some vegetarians may include eggs and dairy products while others

Table 2 Summary of regional diets of the main Asian groups in Britain by country of origin

	Indian Punjab		Gujarat		Pakistan	Bangladesh
	Sikhs	Hindus	Hindus	Moslems	Moslems	Moslems
Main staple cereal	chapattis	chapattis	chapattis or rice	chapattis or rice	chapattis	rice
Main fats	ghee	ghee	groundnut or mustard oil some ghee	groundnut or mustard oil some ghee	ghee or groundnut oil	groundnut or mustard oil a little ghee
Meat and fish	no beef some vegetarians others eat mainly chicken or mutton no fish	no beef mostly vegetarians no fish	no beef mostly vegetarians some fish	no pork halal meat only (usually chicken or mutton) little if any fish	no pork halal meat only (usually chicken or mutton) little fish	no pork halal meat only (usually chicken or mutton) a lot of fresh or dried fish

Eggs	not a major part of the diet	not eaten by strict vegetarians	not eaten by strict vegetarians	usually hard-boiled, fried, or omelette	usually hard-boiled, fried, or omelette	few – usually hard-boiled, fried, or omelette (in curries)
Dairy products	very important: milk yoghurt curd cheese	very important: milk yoghurt curd cheese	important: milk yoghurt	fairly: important milk yoghurt	fairly important: milk yoghurt	few: milk
Pulses	major source of protein	major source of protein	major source of protein	important	important	important
Vegetables and fruit	curries occasional salad fresh fruit	curries occasional salad fresh fruit	curries occasional salad fresh fruit	curries occasional salad fresh fruit	curries occasional salad fresh fruit	curries occasional salad fresh fruit

Note: Asian families in East Africa ate a diet largely based on the area of the subcontinent from which they emigrated.

follow a completely vegan diet. Fast days are common and may follow different patterns, from total elimination of food to a day where foods are restricted to those which are considered 'pure' e.g. rice and fruit. The caste system also dictates who can prepare and share food.

The traditional staple cereal among Gujaratis is millet, but wheat flour is more frequently used to make chapattis, puris and parathas (types of bread) in the UK. Ghee or oil is used in cooking and a variety of pulses/lentils (dhals) and vegetables are eaten.

Sikhs

The Sikh community primarily originates from the Indian Punjab. Their religion, Sikhism, draws upon both Hindu and Moslem traditions. Consequently vegetarianism is not uncommon and Sikhs who do eat meat will not eat beef or pork. However, non-vegetarian Sikhs will usually consume mutton, poultry, fish, eggs and dairy products such as yoghurt, buttermilk and panir (homemade cheese). The staple cereal for Punjabis is wheat. Although rice is eaten it is less important in the diet. Ghee is commonly used in cooking, although the use of oil is now becoming more frequent.

Moslems

Although the Indian community includes a few Gujarati Moslems, the majority of Moslems in this country come from Pakistan and Bangladesh. The Bangladeshi community originates primarily from the Sylhet district and tends to be more homogeneous in cultural and socio-economic terms than other groups. They are the most recent immigrants to the UK.

Islam provides directives regulating all aspects of life, including food preparation and eating. Food laws are derived from the Koran, which forbids the consumption of alcohol, pork, carnivorous animals and some birds. Poultry and fish with scales are permitted. All meat consumed must be from animals killed by ritual slaughter (Halal). Utensils which have come into contact with pork or pork products cannot be used for cooking. During the lunar month of Ramadhan all Moslems should fast between sunrise and sunset. Those who are ill, pregnant, or on a journey may be excused; provided that they make up the days of fasting on another occasion. Since it is more convenient to fast when the rest of the family is fasting, pregnant women may choose not to take up this dispensation and so may fast during their pregnancy. Menstruating women are forbidden from fasting during Ramadhan. The Koran also advocates that children should be breast-fed up to the age of two years.

The staple food for Pakistani Moslems is the chapatti, made from wheat. Meat, vegetables and dhals are also eaten. Bangladeshi Moslems place a much greater emphasis on fish.

Patterns of change

Some Asian communities have maintained their traditions more strongly than others. At the more non-traditional end of the spectrum are those who came from East Africa. Punjabi Sikhs and Gujarati Hindus show more influence of tradition, while Pakistanis and Bangladeshis are likely to have maintained their traditions most strongly. Clearly, this a broad generalisation and within each community there are individuals who follow traditional patterns more or less strictly.

This diversity is also seen in eating patterns. Those who are socially isolated from the majority Caucasian population are more likely to eat traditional foods, e.g. the old, people with poor language skills and women whose activities outside the home are restricted by cultural tradition. Amongst Hindus, more women than men maintain a vegetarian diet, while those following a mixed diet tend to be younger and to consume only small quantities of meat.

The person responsible for food-shopping can also affect the type of foods available within the household. Amongst

Moslems, this task is often carried out by men, who are more inclined to purchase only what is familiar to them, for example, imported vegetables from Asian-owned shops. In the less traditional Sikh and Hindu households, women are generally responsible for food purchases and make a more varied choice. However, frozen or canned vegetables are rarely consumed.

Some evidence suggests a loss of confidence in the nutritional value of a traditional diet as a result of negative attitudes in the wider community. Unfortunately, changes in food habits which do occur may reduce the quality of the diet. For example younger people appear to be increasing their consumption of fizzy drinks, confectionery and fast foods. The extent of this trend, however, has not been thoroughly investigated.

Infant feeding practices

Breast and bottle feeding Studies consistently report lower levels of breast feeding in the UK than in the subcontinent, where it is the traditional method of feeding. The incidence of breast feeding also varies within the Asian community, although it is difficult to make generalisations or to identify trends, as the methodology used varies between studies. East African Asians tend to breast feed for a short period of time, while breast feeding among Punjabi Indians follows a similar pattern to the host community, although girls are less likely to be breast-fed than boys. There is a tendency for more Pakistanis to breast feed and to do so for a longer period of time. A variety of reasons have been identified amongst Bangladeshi women for not practising breast feeding and these include: observation of the high levels of bottle feeding among the Caucasian population living in the same areas; the prestige value attached to bottle feeding, as a western practice; lack of privacy due to overcrowded housing conditions; difficulties in communications with health professionals; and early return to working situations where there are no opportunities for breast feeding.

Introduction of cow's milk and weaning Reports are frequently made of both early and late weaning, and prolonged feeding on cow's milk. It is common for Asian women to change from infant formula to 'doorstep' milk at about 5-6 months of age. Late weaning seems to be more common among children born in the Indian subcontinent, or born to mothers who have only been in the UK for a short time. However, children who are born in this country are more likely to be weaned early. A recent study has also found prolonged use of feeding bottles among Asian infants. Most were still using a bottle at the age of two years, and two-thirds of the milk feeds were sweetened.

Excessive and inappropriate use of commercially prepared baby foods has also aroused concern. Since Moslem mothers will not introduce savoury weaning foods that contain non-halal meat and vegetarian households avoid varieties containing meat altogether, there is a tendency to rely heavily on sweet dessert-type baby foods, often low in protein and iron.

The Afro-Caribbean community: religious and cultural traditions

The majority of Afro-Caribbeans in the UK are Christians and, as a result, their dietary patterns are free from religious influence, but reflect the influence of the colonisers of the Caribbean islands. The diet is therefore based on cereals such as rice, maize and wheat; roots, and tubers such as yams, sweet potatoes, breadfruit and plantain. These are generally consumed with meats such as chicken and goat, both fresh and salted fish (e.g. salt fish and ackee (a vegetable) is a traditional favourite). Dishes are well seasoned with herbs and spices and frequently eaten in the form of stews. Homemade soup is also very popular.

Within the Afro-Caribbean community, a minority are Rastafarians and follow the dietary regulations with varying degrees of strictness. The most orthodox eat only 'I-tal' or 'natural' foods. Processed and preserved foods are excluded, since food additives are believed to pollute the body and soul. Canned food is also avoided. Meat, poultry, eggs and dairy products are unacceptable, while alcohol and salt are prohibited. A second group of Rastafarians, who are drawn mainly from a more educated or professional section of the population, accept the central tenets of the 'I-tal' code, but consume dairy products, small quantities of scaled fish, and sea-salt and other seasonings. In contrast, there is also a group of socially deprived Rastafarians, often unemployed and without permanent accommodation, who are unlikely to eat regular meals and are unable to follow the dietary code.

Patterns of change

Food consumption patterns in the Afro-Caribbean community have not been investigated to the same extent as those of Asians. However, it seems that while the first generation immigrants were anxious to abandon the traditional diet, regarding it as 'poor people's' food, for the younger generation it represents a statement of identity and culture. Recent surveys suggest the traditional foods remain popular among Afro-Caribbeans. One report from London found that 86% of respondents ate at least one traditional meal each day and of these, three quarters were aged between 29 and 40 years. Similarly in Birmingham a survey found that 31% ate traditional meals almost every day and a further 46% did so between one and three times each week.

Infant feeding practices

Breast and bottle feeding Although few studies of Afro-Caribbean infant-feeding practices have been carried out, the picture which emerges suggests that traditional practices have been retained and over 90% of women may breast feed initially. However, the proportion drops fairly rapidly and exclusive breast feeding is rare.

Introduction of cow's milk and weaning Early weaning seems to be common. The introduction of semi-solid foods like banana and home-made cornmeal porridge at the age of one month has been reported. At three months, as many as 45% may have been introduced to solids, often to commercially available cereals, with a greater variety of traditional foods being introduced later.

Nutritional implications

The available information suggests that diets differ not only within the Asian and Afro-Caribbean communities, but also between these minority ethnic groups and the Caucasian population. Except for a few conditions caused by specific dietary deficiencies, there is no evidence that ethnic differences in dietary patterns are responsible for ethnic differences in rates of diseases such as hypertension, coronary heart disease and diabetes. The problems which arise amongst various sections of these communities are now considered.

Pregnant women

When the maternal diet is inadequate, the additional demands of pregnancy are often considered to put at risk the health of women and their unborn babies. As a result, pregnant women are frequently considered to be a 'vulnerable group' requiring special attention in their own right, as well as serving as a broader indication of dietary adequacy.

Nutrient intakes

A number of studies examining the adequacy of the diets of pregnant Asian women suggest that intakes of some nutrients may be lower than those of Caucasian women. However, the results have not always been consistent. Although energy intakes below recommended levels have been reported for all groups, some studies have shown differences between Sikhs, Pakistanis, Hindus and Bangladeshis while others have not. One study has shown the protein intakes of vegan Hindu women to be significantly lower than those of non-vegetarians, while another study found higher protein intakes among Hindus when compared with other groups. A study carried out in Birmingham reported that Sikhs had the highest intakes of energy and most nutrients, while Bangladeshi women had the lowest. However all groups in this study had below the recommended intakes of zinc, copper, vitamin B_{12}, riboflavin and vitamin D.

Low birth weight

The clinical significance of these findings is unclear. Although studies in the UK have consistently shown that babies born to Asian women are lighter on average by 150-350g than those born to Caucasian women in the same area, it is uncertain whether this is due to genetic factors or to poor maternal nutrition. The trend towards increasing birth weights over a period of ten years would suggest that genetic factors are not the major cause of these differences. Changes in factors such as longer birth intervals, fewer teenage pregnancies and better nutrition may all play a part. Differences have also been noted between groups, with Sikh infants being significantly longer and heavier than Moslem or Hindu infants, although the reason for this is unclear.

Vitamin D deficiency

Studies suggest that signs of Vitamin D deficiency are evident in Asian women during pregnancy and that if left untreated there is a greater risk of neonatal hypocalcaemia and rickets. The benefits of supplementation with vitamin D (as recommended by the Department of Health for all women during pregnancy) have been demonstrated for Asian women.

Infants and children

A nutritionally adequate diet is essential for health and normal growth and consequently the nutritional status of infants and children is particularly important in any consideration of nutrition in ethnic minority groups. However, there is a considerable lack of information available, due in part to the methodological difficulties involved in gaining accurate nutritional data concerning this age group in general.

Nutrient intakes

At present, there is no information available concerning the nutrient intakes of Afro-Caribbean infants and children, and information about Asian children is limited to infants and pre-school children. There is also a lack of consistency in the findings of these studies, although energy intakes below the recommended levels have been found in all groups.

A study of infants at 3, 6, 9, 12 and 24 months of age found the mean intake of protein among Asian children to be lower than Caucasians, but above the recommended levels, except at 3 and 12 months. In contrast, between 45-75% of Bangladeshi children have been reported to consume less than the recommended amount of protein between the ages of 6 months and 4 years. The same studies reported adequate calcium and vitamin C intakes, with the main nutrient deficiencies being of vitamin D and iron amongst intakes of infants aged one year and over.

Growth

The diversity of the minority ethnic population, and question marks over the appropriateness of British growth standards, make it difficult to interpret differences in growth patterns among these children. However, there is evidence to suggest that despite low birth weight, Asian children grow just as well as Caucasians.

A study of Asian and Caucasian children, matched for sex and socio-economic status, found the growth patterns were similar in the two groups throughout the first two years. However, both groups were below the 50th centile of Tanner and Whitehouse UK growth standards, with a tendency for Asians to be smaller than Caucasians. Bangladeshi infants up to the age of 18 months have also been reported to be consistently below the 50th centile. In contrast, a study of Punjabi children found they tended to remain above 90 per cent of the Tanner 50th centile for bodyweight during the first two years.

Growth of Caucasian children and those from minority ethnic groups have been monitored, between the ages of 5 and 11 years, as part of the National Study of Health and Growth. Afro-Caribbean children were consistently above the 50th centile at most ages. However, within the Afro-Caribbean group there was greater variation in stature, short statue corresponding to low socio-economic status. Within the Asian community, the Gujarati children were the shortest, followed by the Pakistani children, with the Punjabi Sikh children closest to the 50th centile. In most cases there were no differences between vegetarians and non-vegetarians, with the exception of Pakistani girls, where those who were vegetarians were significantly shorter. Among the Asian groups in general, lower levels of maternal education and greater household overcrowding were associated with smaller stature.

Studies also show different patterns of fat distribution. It seems that Afro-Caribbean children have the lowest amounts of subcutaneous fat. Although the total body fat of Asian and Caucasian children appears to be the same, Asian children have bigger fat deposits on the trunk and smaller deposits on the limbs than Caucasians.

Ethnic variation has been estimated to account for 5% of the variation in children's height. The larger variation in height of Afro-Caribbean children suggests that there is potential for increased growth within this group.

Anaemia

Iron deficiency anaemia has been observed in Afro-Caribbean children since the early 1960s. However, iron deficiency appears to be most prevalent among children from the Asian community, especially Moslem children. In all groups, higher prevalence is associated with poorer socio-economic conditions. Although the role of prolonged breast feeding in this problem has been disputed, it is probable that the early introduction and excessive intake of unfortified cow's milk in Asian children may result in iron deficiency in those whose iron status is already low.

Vitamin D deficiency and rickets

Rickets (a childhood disease causing softening and deformation of the bones due to deficiency of vitamin D and calcium) was first reported among Asian children in the early 1960s. In the following period to the mid 1980s, evidence indicated that the incidence of rickets was in decline, and at a low level in 1985. Cases have also been reported from the Afro-Caribbean community, but these have been less common.

There have been many studies into the cause of rickets among Asians. Although much is now known, further work is needed. Susceptibility to rickets appears to be related to a number of risk factors, the most important of which are dietary. High risk is associated with diets high in phytate (a substance found in whole grain cereals which binds with minerals so that they cannot be absorbed) and fibre, with little or no food of animal origin. Such a diet is likely to increase the need for calcium and vitamin D, and foods of animal origin are considered to be protective. Other risk factors are a low exposure to sunlight, due to poor living conditions and customs of clothing and seclusion, and a darker skin colour.

Adults

Nutrient intake

Although there have been no large scale nutritional surveys in the adult Asian and Afro-Caribbean population, some dietary data is available from studies investigating the factors contributing to excess rates of heart disease in the Asian population. The results of these studies indicated that the Asian men (Gujarati) had lower energy intakes than Caucasians with similar total fat intakes as a percentage of dietary energy (38%). The P/S ratio was substantially higher among Asians than Caucasians, while intakes of iron and fibre were similar.

Anaemia

Nutritional megaloblastic anaemia, a relatively rare type of anaemia, resulting from vitamin B_{12} deficiency has been associated with a strict vegetarian diet. Studies indicate that vitamin B_{12} deficiency is predominantly a problem in vegetarian Hindu women. There is evidence that the incidence of nutritional megaloblastic anaemia from vitamin B_{12} is declining as a result of changing dietary patterns among subsequent generations of Asians in the UK.

Iron deficiency anaemia is considered to be widespread. In a study of Punjabi women, 32% had serum iron levels below 10µmol/l.

Vitamin D deficiency and osteomalacia

Vitamin D deficiency first aroused concern in the early 1960s following a report on rickets and osteomalacia (a bone disorder in adults resulting from vitamin D and calcium deficiency) among Asian immigrants in Glasgow. Subsequent studies have confirmed vitamin D deficiency in the Asian population, with estimates of prevalence ranging from 3.5% to 38%. A steady, small number of cases of osteomalacia in Asian women continues to be reported.

Results from a study in which the vitamin D status of a group of healthy Asians was compared with that of a control group of healthy Caucasians, indicated that 22% of the Asians had low serum vitamin D (25-OHD) levels while none of the Caucasians did. Gujaratis had higher levels than Punjabis, but there was no relationship between serum concentration of vitamin D (25-OHD) and vegetarian diet or length of residence in the UK.

Coronary heart disease and hypertension

In England and Wales between 1979-83, mortality from coronary heart disease (CHD) among Asian men and women was higher than the national average. This contrasted with low CHD mortality in Afro-Caribbeans. Further studies suggest that high rates are shared by all Asians, irrespective of geographical origins or socio-economic group. Rates of CHD amongst Asian migrants in other parts of the world are also high.

Analysis of conventional risk factors suggests that while hypertension, diet, serum cholesterol and stress are important in Asian migrants, they do not completely explain the high incidence of CHD among Asians. However, the high rates of non-insulin-dependent diabetes may make a significant contribution and the role of stress is largely unexplored.

To illustrate, while heavy smoking among Bangladeshi men has been reported, General Household Survey data suggest that smoking rates are lower among Asians than the general population. Studies of Bangladeshis in East London and Gujaratis in North West London found mean plasma cholesterol levels significantly lower than those of Caucasians. Diet does not appear to provide a satisfactory explanation either. Two recent studies have found Gujarati Hindus to have low dietary intakes of saturated fat and cholesterol and high P/S ratios, although total fat intake is close to the national average. However, this group is predominantly vegetarian and sources of dietary saturated fat are restricted to dairy products. This is not the case for non-vegetarian groups, for which there is no published data. The suggestion that cholesterol oxides in ghee might be a factor has not been supported by later work. In addition ghee is not used universally by all the different sub-groups within the Asian community, yet all of them experience the same high risk of CHD.

In contrast to the Asian population, mortality data show a high incidence of hypertension and stroke amongst the Afro-Caribbean community. There is evidence to show that hypertension affects urban black populations all over the world, not just in the UK. Although it has been suggested that this may be linked to high salt intakes, clear evidence to support this view is not available. However, this does not mean that control of obesity and salt intake does not have a role to play in prevention.

Diabetes

Non-insulin dependent diabetes is a common problem among both the Afro-Caribbean and Asian communities. A survey of the prevalence of diabetes in Southall found diabetes to be almost four times more common in Asians than among Caucasians. It is possible that diets high in sugar and low in fibre and starch increase the risk of developing diabetes. Diets high in sugar and refined carbohydrates have been reported amongst Asian diabetics. However, there is no evidence that Asians and Afro-Caribbeans consume more or less fibre than the national average. It has recently been suggested that insulin resistance associated with obesity may account for the high prevalence of diabetes in the Asian community. It would seem, therefore, that control of obesity should be encouraged in Asians.

Obesity

Although little data is available on this, at least one study has reported higher prevalence of obesity among Asians when compared with Afro-Caribbeans and Caucasians.

Conclusions

It must be emphasised that the traditional diets of Asians and Afro-Caribbeans in the UK are, in general, not only compatible with adequate nutrition, but in some aspects closer to current dietary recommendations than Caucasian diets (e.g. fat and fibre). Nonetheless, within any community, there may exist groups who are particularly vulnerable to malnutrition. Poor housing, low incomes, poor working conditions, unemployment and racism may all contribute to inadequate nutrition among those trying to maintain traditional diets.

In addition to the problems of 'at-risk' groups such as infants, pre-school children and pregnant women there are other groups which need to be considered. Recent migrants to the UK may have particular problems in adapting traditional practices.

It is important also to emphasise the heterogeneity of these communities. Among the Asian population, cultural, religious, and linguistic diversity are combined with varying degrees of traditionalism. Similarly, Afro-Caribbeans in the UK come from different islands in the West Indies with different traditions. At the same time a new generation, born in this country, is growing up with changing patterns of eating.

From this review it is clear that information on the state of nutrition of Britain's minority ethnic population is both scarce and patchy. Most published data has been concerned with a number of 'special problems' such as rickets, low birth weight, anaemia and infant feeding. No information is currently available about nutrition among elderly members of minority communities, yet this is clearly an area which will become increasingly important. There has also been a heavy emphasis on inquiries among the Asian community in contrast to the lack of nutritional information concerning Afro-Caribbeans. Similarly, there is very little nutritional information available for other minority ethnic groups. For these reasons the need for further research is heavily emphasised in the ideas for action which follow.

Nutrition education

1 Nutrition education should promote the positive aspects of traditional diets.

2 Where appropriate, minority ethnic cultures, foods and diets should be included in the teaching curriculum of home economics, catering, dietetics and all health related training.

3 Given the heterogeneity of the Asian and Afro-Caribbean communities, resource materials should be appropriate to the specific community being addressed.

4 Education concerning food selection must take account of varying patterns of responsibility for food purchase.

5 Relevant and acceptable, multi-lingual information, based on the views of ethnic minority communities and the advice of those working with them, should be provided.

Research areas

6 Studies of nutrient intake and nutritional status of children, adolescents and adults and the elderly should be a research priority.

7 Studies of eating habits and factors influencing change, particularly in groups such as young people born in the UK, need to be undertaken.

8 Further research is necessary concerning lifestyle and perceptions of health to ensure that nutritional advice given is likely to be culturally acceptable and effective.

Further reading

Abraham, R., Campbell Brown, M., Haines, A.P., North, W.R.S., Hainsworth, V., McFayden, I.R. (1985) Diet during pregnancy in an Asian community in Britain – energy, protein, zinc, copper, fibre and calcium. *Human Nutrition: Applied Nutrition* **39A**, 23-25.

Abraham, R., Campbell Brown, M., North, W.R.S., McFayden, I.R. (1987) Diets of Asian pregnant women in Harrow: iron and vitamins. *Human Nutrition: Applied Nutrition* **41A**, 164-173.

Balarajan, R., Adelstein, A.M., Bulusu, L., Shulela, V. (1984) Patterns of mortality among immigrants to England and Wales from the Indian subcontinent. *British Medical Journal* **289**, 1185-1187.

Campbell Brown, M., Ward, R.J., Haines, A.P., North, W.R.S., Abraham, R., McFayden, I.R. (1985) Zinc and copper nutrition in Asian pregnancies – is there evidence for a nutritional deficiency? *British Journal of Obstetrics and Gynaecology* **92**, 875-885.

Chanarin, I., Malkowska, V., O'Hea, A., Rinsler, M.G., Price, A.B. (1985) Megaloblastic anaemia in a vegetarian Hindu community. *Lancet*, **2**, 1168-1172.

Clarson, C.L., Barter, M.J., Marshall, T., Wharton, B.A. (1982) Secular changes in birthweight of Asian babies born in Birmingham. *Archives of Disease in Childhood* **57**, 867-871.

COMA (1980) Rickets and Osteomalacia. *DHSS Report on Health and Social Subjects* **19**, HMSO, London.

Coronary Prevention Group. (1986) *Coronary Heart Disease and Asians in Britain*. London Confederation of Indian Organisations.

D'Souza, S.W., Lakani, P., Waters, H.M., Boardman, K.M., Clinkotai, K.I. (1987) Iron deficiency in ethnic minorities: association with dietary fibre and phytate. *Early Human Development* 15, 103-111.

Eaton, P.M. (1982) What do Asian women in Birmingham eat during pregnancy? *Proceedings of the Nutrition Society* 41, 257-259.

Erhardt, P. (1986) Iron deficiency in young Bradford children from different ethnic groups. *British Medical Journal* 292, 90-93.

Ginndulis, H., Scott, P.H., Belton, N.R., Wharton, B.A. (1986) An association of anaemia with poor vitamin C status in otherwise adequately nourished Asian toddlers: a case for combined prophylaxis. *Proceedings of the Nutrition Society* 45, 122A.

Harris, R.J., Armstrong, D., Ali, R., Loynes, A. (1983) Nutritional survey of Bangladeshi children aged under 5 years in the London Borough of Tower Hamlets. *Archives of Disease in Childhood* 58, 428-432.

Hill, S.E. (1990) *More than Rice and Peas: Guidelines to improve food provision for black and ethnic minorities in Britain*. The Food Commission, London.

Hunt, S.P., O'Riorodan, J.L.H., Windo, J., Truswell, A.S. (1976) Vitamin D status in different subgroups of British Asians. *British Medical Journal* 2, 1351-1354.

Jones, V.M. (1987) Current infant weaning practices within the Bangladeshi community in the London Borough of

Tower Hamlets. *Human Nutrition: Applied Nutrition* **41A**, 349-352.

Marmot, M.G. (1984) Immigrant Mortality in England and Wales 1970-78. *OPCS Studies of Medical Population Subjects* **47**. London HMSO.

Mather, H.M., Keen, H. (1985) The Southall Diabetes Survey: prevalence of known diabetes in Asians and Europeans. *British Medical Journal* **291**, 1081-1084.

Matthews, J.H., Wood, J.K. (1987) Megaloblastic anaemia in vegetarian Asians. *Clinical Laboratory Haematology* **8**, 1-7.

McFayden, I.R., Campbell Brown, M., Abraham, R., North, W.R.S., Haines, A.P. (1984) Factors affecting birthweight in Hindus, Moslems and Europeans. *British Journal of Obstetrics and Gynaecology* **91**, 968-972.

McKeigue, P.M., Adelstein, A.M., Shipley, M.J., Riermersma, R.A., Marmot, M.G., Hunt, S.P., Butler, S.M., Turner, P.R. (1985) Diet and risk factors for coronary heart disease in Asians in North West London. *Lancet* **2**, 1086-1089.

McKeigue, P.M., Marmot, M.G. (1988) Mortality from coronary heart disease in Asian communities. *British Medical Journal* **297**, 903.

McNeil, G. (1985) Birthweight, feeding practices and weight-for-age for Punjabi children in the UK and in the rural Punjab. *Human Nutrition: Clinical Nutrition* **39C**, 69-72.

Miller, G.J., Kotecha, S., Wilkinson, W.H., Wilkes, H., Stirling, Y., Sanders, T.A.B., Broadhurst, A., Allison, J., Meade, T.W. (1988) Dietary and other characteristics relevant for coronary heart disease in men of Indian, West Indian and European descent in London. *Atherosclerosis* **70**, 63-72.

Roberts, P.D., James, H., Petrie, A., Morgan, J.O., Hoffbrand, A.V. (1973) Vitamin B_{12} status in pregnancy among immigrants to Britain. *British Medical Journal*, **3**, 67-70.

Robertson, I., Glekin, B.M., Henderson, J., McIntosh, W.B., Lachani, A., Dunningan, M.G. (1982) Nutritional deficiencies in ethnic minorities in the UK. *Proceedings of the Nutrition Society* **41**, 243-255.

Shaunak, S., Colston, K., Ang, L., Patel, S.P., Maxwell, J.D. (1985) Vitamin D deficiency in adult British Hindu Asians: a family disorder. *British Medical Journal* **291**, 1166-1169.

Silman, A., Loysen, E., Graff, W., Stramek, M. (1985) High dietary fat intake and cigarette smoking as risk factors for ischaemic heart disease in Bangladeshi male immigrants in East London. *Journal of Epidemiological and Community Health* **39**, 301-305.

Simmons, D., Williams, D.R.R., Powell, M.J. (1989) Prevalence of diabetes in a predominantly Asian community: Preliminary findings of Coventry Diabetes Study. *British Medical Journal* **298**, 18-20.

Stockley, L., Broadhurst, A.J., Kotecha, S. (1987) Nutrient and food intakes in Caucasian and Gujarati men in North London. *Proceedings of the Nutrition Society* **46**, 7A.

Warrington, S., Storey, D.M. (1989) Comparative studies of Asian and Caucasian children. 1 Growth. *European Journal of Clinical Nutrition* **42**, 61-67.

Warrington, S., Storey, D.M. (1988) Comparative studies of Asian and Caucasian children, 2 nutrition, feeding practices and health. *European Journal of Clinical Nutrition* **42**, 69-80.

Wharton, P.A., Eaton, P.M., Wharton, B.A. (1984) Subethnic variation in the diets of Moslems, Sikh, and Hindu pregnant women at Sorrento Maternity Hospital, Birmingham. *British Journal of Nutrition* **52**, 469-476.